# One Potato Chip at a Time
### *The Fat Guy's <u>Honest</u> Diet Guide*

Charles Pluckhahn

Snowden Road Books—White Salmon, WA
ISBN: 979-8-218-33551-9
Library of Congress Control Number: 2023924010
Title: *One Potato Chip at a Time: The Fat Guy's Honest Diet Guide*
Author: Charles Pluckhahn
Digital distribution | 2023
Paperback | 2023


charliewp@protonmail.com

# Dedication

This book would not exist but for Thomas Harwood, one of my cousins, who provided encouragement and a brief critique at just the right time. Thank you, Tom.

And thanks to the L.A. Fitness chain of gyms for introducing its members, including me, to the Harris-Benedict equation, and for having the corporate integrity to correct a transcription mistake that I found, at material expense to the company and to the benefit of the membership.

# Table of Contents

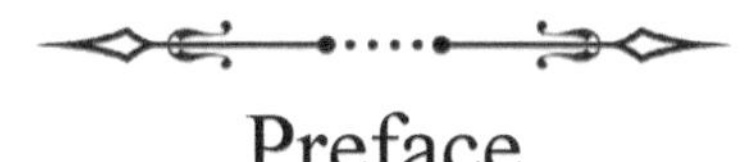

# Preface

Congratulations for picking up my book, and now *your* book!

*"First you've got to get the facts. Then you've got to face the facts."*

*-Paul Cabot, founder of State Street Research & Management Co., which made Harvard University into the financial giant it is today.*

This book will not make you rich or smart, but it will show you how to lose weight, and look and feel better. Keep going, and you will learn the facts you need to make the change you desire. It will not be easy, but it will be honest and straightforward: no gimmicks, no magic, no shortcuts, no evasions, no secrets – including the latest popular appetite suppressing drugs. (See Chapters 7 and 10 for more about that near-fraud.)

This book is built on well-established, old-school science and its application in the real world. Oh, and this is how I lost 40 pounds. It works, and you are going to see exactly how and why it does.

*"Don't tell me what I want to hear. Tell me what I need to hear."*

That is what I aim to do here. What happens now is

your call. But here you are, reading this. Please take it seriously. It could change your life. I did not write this book to make any money – hardly any books do. I wrote this in hopes that my experience, and the facts I picked up along the way, can help you, the valued reader who stumbled across this little guide.

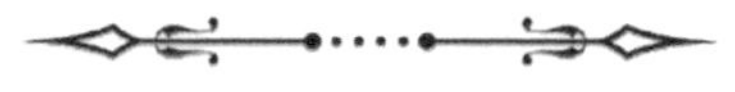

# Chapter 1
## *Santa, How Did I Get So Fat?*

It's Christmas, and you are struggling. Your pants don't fit and your shirt collar won't button. You stand in front of the mirror, grab hold of that belly roll, and manage to suck in your gut long enough to cinch your belt. Again. Oh yeah, you've been here before. So have I. You even have that red line around your waist to prove it. You tell yourself for the 50th time: I have to do something. But what?

Ten years ago, we started jogging. It didn't do anything but make our shins and joints sore. Not to mention that running is a boring pain in the ass, truly one of the most overrated forms of recreation ever invented. But we tried. We switched to low-fat foods. It didn't do a damn thing, but we tried. We got gym memberships with no results because we didn't really know what we were doing. But we tried. Maybe you even bought a bicycle – I thought about it -- but you are still fat and now you run red lights and stop signs. Just last week you were almost flattened by a truck. Now what? Try harder?

You do need to keep trying, but effectively. And the first step to effectiveness is to stop insulting yourself. Really, guy, just quit that! It doesn't help at all. ***This is an engineering problem, not a morality play.*** Chances are that you did not gain 50 pounds by eating cherry pies in the middle of the night. Nope, you got fat 8 calories at a time. It blew my mind to find out, but it's true. Until you wrap your head around that reality, you won't get anywhere. So, guy, let's get moving and start by having a truly honest talk about all this.

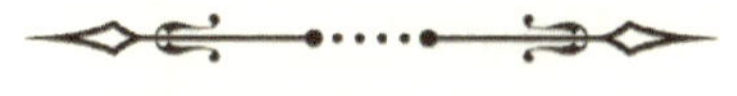

# Chapter 2
### *Who Needs another Diet Book?*

You do! But this chapter's title is why I almost did not publish this book. Not only are there plenty of these diet books—*understatement of the century*—but I offer only research, ethics, and personal experience. Not being part of Weight Loss Inc., I certainly don't have the money for infomercials, nor the backing of major publishers with insider connections.

But consider this: Weight Loss Inc. has been around for decades. They must be doing something right, even if it's simply making piles of money. Far be it for me to argue with that. But in the meantime, according to the Centers for Disease Control, obesity has gone from 13% to 43% of the U.S. population in the past 60 years. Heck of a job you've done, Weight Watchers, Nutrisystems, Jenny Craig, and others. With friends like you, who really needs enemies?

Here is the worst: Talk to fat people and you will quickly learn how many blame their situation on a uniquely slow metabolism. And there is another category of rampant misinformation. It blames overweight on what Michael Pollan, the famed nutrition author, termed the latest "food villain." Is it sugar? Is it salt? How about gluten, chemtrails, Roundup, Aspartame, or other "toxins?" Anything but the fork. Oh God, not the fork!

Here are some things this book does *not* do:

**Treat everyone the same**:

This book aims at otherwise healthy, middle-aged people who want to lose 30 or 50 or 70 pounds. If you wonder whether or not your health can handle it, talk to a doctor first. If you have a chronic health issue, or are severely obese, you'll need more specialized help. Chances are that a good deal of that help will be broadly congruent with what's here, yet you will need more assistance than I can provide.

By the way, I wrote for middle-aged men for the sole reason that they are an under-served group. There is no reason why this can't work for women. Or older folks. Or the young; in fact, this book would make a great gift for a high school or college kid to educate them about metabolism. If I had known about it in my 20s, I'd have avoided some mistakes later on. I address women in some detail in Chapter 5, and cover metabolism and age in several chapters.

**Lie or mislead**:

Ecclesiastes (the Bible guy) had a great point about there being nothing new under the sun. This book combines pre-existing elements – which, incidentally, is true of most products and services. Contrary to what's implied by those infomercials, there are no effortless solutions. There are no miracles. Those are dishonest, and this is an "Honest Diet Guide." But there is a simple, methodical, scientific approach that will yield results – and this is it.

**Be your therapist:**

Too many diet books go there, but the only "therapy" here is to advise you to forgive your ignorance about metabolism and try not to beat yourself up for being fat. Trust me, I am not against therapy, but I have no skill at it. If you take that route, I think you will eventually come back here for the mechanics of weight loss. This is a "how to" book, nothing more.

**Overwhelm you**:

My goal is to be clear, concise, and correct, so as not to occupy any more of your valuable time than I have to. But please don't mistake my breezy, somewhat irreverent style for a lack of seriousness. There is nothing casual here. I have listed sources and citations for this book's relevant claims in the appendices, along with other supplementary information.

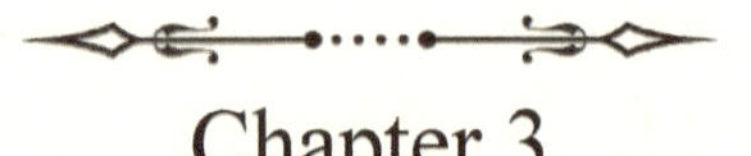

# Chapter 3
## *Metabolism, the Cornerstone*

James Arthur Harris and Francis Gano Benedict, a pair of researchers working with the Carnegie Institution of Washington, D.C. wrote the comprehensive, indispensable, and thoroughly mind-numbing *A Biometric Study of Basal Metabolism in Man.* It was published in 1919. What?! You mean to tell me that the guts of this book have been around since then? Yep, no fooling: ***This science is now more than a century old. More people should know about it, and that is why the world needs yet another diet book. Or at least this one.***

Harris and Benedict were interested in how many calories someone needs to maintain their weight. Why did they care? Simple answer: World War I was on while they were working, and they were interested in food rationing. In later years, their research helped managers of custodial institutions – hospitals, boarding schools, colleges, prisons, and the military – figure out how much food to serve. Harris and Benedict used multiple regression analysis, a powerful statistical technique, to identify and measure what influences someone's weight. The computer spreadsheet makes it pretty easy to perform multiple regressions today. They did it manually back then. Ugh. And thank you!

In the end, they isolated the following: Whether or not someone is ambulatory or bedridden, and their sex, height, weight, and age. They even came up with a formula. If you know those numbers and plug them into the formula, you can establish a "calorie budget" that will stabilize your weight. Even though it was not aimed at taking off pounds, the Harris-Benedict Equation can be used to construct an effective diet program, especially when combined with other longstanding research on exercise and nutrition.

**I got fat eight calories at a time? And you're not lying?**

I swear on a stack that am telling you the God's honest truth, and I will prove it. Seriously, that is almost certainly what happened, at least in the beginning before you gave up. Now let me tell you why. Be patient. Keep reading, and you will see.

Part of Harris and Benedict's groundbreaking work was a *crucial* discovery that *everyone* ought to know about: Metabolism declines with age. As you get older, you need to eat a little less every year. Not a lot less, but just a little. After you are 25 or so, a man's calorie budget declines by 8.4 calories a day, every year, as his metabolism naturally slows down.

That's next to nothing in any one year, but how about a decade? Eat like you did at 25 when you are 35, and that's 3,066 extra calories a year. But that's only an extra slice of bread every two weeks! You are going to see how much it actually matters, but still: *No one can blame you for not noticing.* In any case: You did not pig out. You ate normally. And that is why you have (and why I had) that embarrassing muffin top. It's why you have that red line around your waist from tightening your belt too far.

***How much damage can "an extra slice of bread every two weeks" do? Brace yourself for some bad news, maybe even shockingly bad.***

A pound of fat provides 3,500 calories of energy. If you eat more calories than your body requires, and you do not jog or starve it off, your body will turn it into fat. Ergo, if you eat the way you did at 25 when you're 35, and your exercise habits have not changed, you will be gaining fat at a rate of 8 or 9 pounds per decade. Keep it up for 10 more years, and you'll put on another 17 or 18 pounds. All because you ate as much as you got older as you did when you were younger.

And that's not the whole story. Chances are that you started eating *more* when you left school and started earning money. You've probably been working longer hours, and have exercised *less* than you used to. So you didn't gain 25 pounds, but maybe 40 or 50 or 60 pounds.

As the weight added up, we denied it at first. Then we fought it with jogging, gym memberships, sporadic fad diets – you name it. Which did not work the way we wanted them to. Why? Because we didn't know anything about metabolism. Guy, don't beat yourself up! When was the last time anyone mentioned it? No one told us. Take heart! Now you have this book. Wow, who knew? Harris and Benedict, that's who. And now you will know, too.

More truth: Our unfocused efforts weren't completely in vain. They did keep us from becoming morbidly obese, and that's worth a lot. Yet here you are, on Christmas Day, wondering if you will be able to buckle your pants. "Not weighing 400 pounds" seems like cold comfort, no? In fact, doesn't it seem to get harder and harder to avoid that disaster? Of course it does! Why? Because your metabolism is declining as you get older. It is perfectly normal, but it makes you feel like you are forever pushing a rock uphill. Sometimes you just want to give up. Sound familiar?

Hang in there! Now you know how it happened. You did not get fat because you are a pig. You did not get fat because your metabolism is out of whack. You got fat because your metabolism is normal, but you did not know what a normal metabolism looks like. The occasional corn dog at the state fair notwithstanding, chances are that you got fat one potato chip at a time. You didn't realize that you need to gradually reduce your food consumption as you get older. It is that simple. Really. Your fault? No, it is not. You did not know. Now you do.

Okay, so it was a bag of chips, a pretzel, and an ice cream cone. Whatever. The point stands: ***You did not get fat by stuffing yourself all the time, but rather by constantly eating a little too much.*** And now I will tell you how to throw it into reverse.

This being a factual book, I refuse to lie and tell you it will be easy. You will not lose 25 pounds in a month, or whatever some shyster on cable TV is promising. But if you follow this program to the letter, you *will* lose that roll. And maybe you will tell others to find a copy of the book that told you the truth and showed you the way. Please?

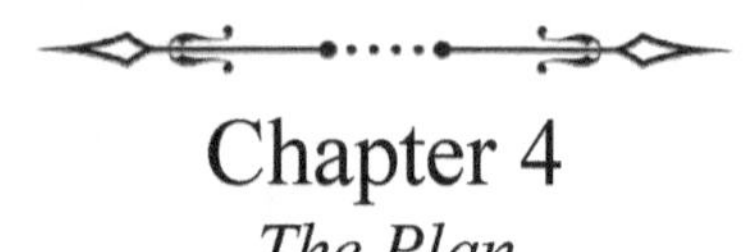

# Chapter 4
## *The Plan*

1. Find your baseline calorie budget.

2. Establish a useful exercise program, and track how many calories you burn.

3. Add 1 and 2, and that is your new "horizon," meaning the calorie intake by which you will neither gain nor lose weight.

4. Deduct 750 calories a day to lose 1-1/2 pounds a week

**"Your Baseline Calorie Budget"**

Using regression analysis, Harris and Benedict established an equation for determining your baseline. At this writing, Cornell University – among others – maintains an excellent calculator that you can use to do it the easy way. Why Cornell? Because their Department of Physiology & Biophysics has a longstanding reputation as one of the world's best. The link is immediately below, but we all know how quickly things change on the internet, so I have reprinted the equation in this book's Appendix A. https://tinyurl.com/hbcornell

**"A Useful Exercise Program"**

For exercise to contribute to weight loss, you should

perform a cardiovascular training routine for 45 uninterrupted minutes. Maintain a heart rate of 80% of a theoretical maximum, determined by subtracting your age from the number 220. Look, guy, I did not make this up. I don't do that. In the appendix, there is a link to a National Institutes of Health paper on the subject.

If you are 50 years old, your "maximum" heart rate is 220 beats per minute minus 50, or 170. Your workout heart rate (the one to maintain for 45 minutes) is 80% of 170, or 136. Here is where a gym membership really helps. Today's treadmills, bikes, elliptical machines, and stair climbers are computerized and give heart rate readouts. They allow you to dial in the level of resistance that will cause your heart to beat at the required rate, and they will tell you how many calories you burned during your session.

To amp this up, perhaps after a few weeks to get used to everything, you can try "interval training," in which you go back and forth between 60%-70% of maximum and (briefly) to 90%-100%. I did it, and found it punishing. But it is also a renowned fat burner. Past that, there is more good news: ***You do not need to jog***. If you are in your 20s or 30s, a stair-climbing machine will do it. If you are older than that, a treadmill, elliptical machine, or stationary bicycle is enough. After your joints thank you, then you can thank me. You're welcome!

If you exercise outside of a gym, you can consult the list in the appendix for the calorie expenditures from exercise. You will need to measure your heart rate and sustain the effort without interruption, so do not fast-walk a course with busy streets to cross. From experience: It can be considerably harder than you might imagine to maintain the required heart rate outside of a gym. However you do it: ***There are no shortcuts. I am not lying to you, so do not lie to yourself! Remember this: There is no deception like self-deception.***

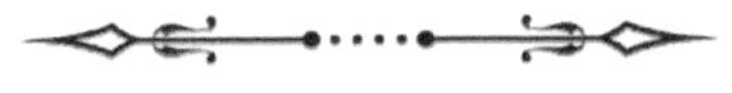

# Chapter 5

## *A Deeper Look at Calories, Metabolism, and Women*

This book is calorie-centric. You must count every last one of them, and conform the total to your specific plan that matches your Harris-Benedict equation. ***Plan calories on a weekly basis. Eat the same number of calories on non-exercise days as you eat on exercise days.*** It will be much simpler, and it will help you avoid the phenomenon of eating too much on exercise days and not adequately counteracting that on non-exercise days.

**Are all calories equal? Mostly, but not entirely:**

1. Sugar is not a "food villain," except for the duration of this program. Sugar is not just desserts. It is also alcohol and refined flour, each of which metabolize into glucose. Why are these so bad on a diet? Because glucose interferes with your body's metabolism of fat. And not by just a little. So that 125-calorie glass of wine, or a 155-calorie beer? Those are very big no-nos, along with white bread and refined flour.

2. Acidic foods burn fat, the leader being grapefruit. There is no small amount of controversy about this. The various studies are inconclusive, so readers will have to make their own call. And there are potential

downsides. The first is that grapefruit, in particular, can interact negatively with some prescription medications. Same thing if you have a problem with acid reflux. So you might need to talk to your doctor first. You might have to avoid this element altogether.

3. Pay attention to fiber. The standard American diet is often quite weak in that area. One excellent source is Wasa brand crackers, which are 100% whole grain. Okay, they taste like cardboard, but the results will be worth it. Another source is citrus. The section "dividers" are pure fiber.

This book's Appendix B gives calorie counts for a list of common foods, and a recipe for a low-cal "power breakfast" – smoked salmon and cream cheese on whole wheat toast and a big-ass glass of carrot-ginger-orange (or apple) juice prepared in a juicer machine as opposed to some filtered, sugary dreck in a bottle or carton at the grocery store. Between the fiber that remains in the juice and the fiber in whole wheat bread, my 600-calorie "power breakfast" is a *superb* source. And it is delicious, which is more than I can say for some other healthy foods. I still eat it on many mornings.

On the fiber front, we cannot forget salads, which you will be eating plenty of in this program. As a general proposition, unrefined "complex" carbs tend to be some of the most filling and less caloric things you can eat, making them excellent tools in a calorie-restricted diet. As you get into this program, you are likely to be surprised by the difference between what you have been eating, and what you should have been eating. I sure as hell was. If you want to open your eyes about what we eat in this country, try this program. Unless you are some sort of food fanatic – which means that you probably would not be reading this anyway – I say that you will never quite eat the same.

Or at least you will be far more aware of what is on that fork. One more thing for now: If you think that my statements are an introduction to a vegan lecture, think again. As I write, the disassembled half of a steer purchased from the rancher and cut by a local butcher, sits in the freezer, just waiting until them steaks are rare, bloody, and sizzling on my plate. Call me names, but I am perfectly comfortable at the top of the food chain. Same goes for trendy vegetables (*kale? Ugh*) or Eastern religion. This is arithmetic, and not a lot else.

Along similar lines, if being overweight is not a morality play, neither is losing weight. If you think, or maybe your significant other thinks, that you are fat because you did not eat organic food, or consumed "toxins," you should stick your fingers in your ears and ignore the kindly advice. Or maybe you could ponder what is really behind it: the notion that you are fat for lack of virtue, and that virtue will make you thinner. Forget that! It is nothing but Old Time Religion with a smiley-face sticker. In lieu of sermons, this program offers a way to reduce your weight and improve your health.

**What About Organic?**

Kill me now, guy, but I'm not sold. Speaking from direct experience, it is quite possible to get organically fat. A specific example appeared while this book was in the publishing stage. There is a purveyor of organic fruit juices that I'd love to name but which I won't because who can afford a lawsuit even if it's groundless? Their stuff is delicious, but I decided to take a closer look at the label and do the arithmetic.

Turned out that my favorite has about 35% more calories (not to mention added "natural flavors") than what I make in my juicer, not to mention no fiber content that I could discern. Where do those calories come from? You got it: the "organic cane sugar" added to the mix, which amounts to about a pound in a gallon jug. Feel virtuous if you'd like, but don't kid yourself about organic.

Oh, and by the way, do you think that organic means no pesticides or herbicides? Think again. Those are just different, much more expensive, and by the account of fruit orchardists who I know and trust, more hazardous to both fruit pickers and consumers. They use them anyway because that's what their export markets demand, but they do chuckle about it. Reader, it's your money and your choice, but do yourself a favor and at least make sure to thoroughly wash any organic produce from the grocery store.

**Some Specific Diet Ideas**

This is an "Honest Diet Guide," so the truth is that it will not be easy. But it will be simple and straightforward. You need information along with your discipline. Between the calories themselves and the need to avoid sugars, you will be reading labels like a hawk.

1. It's not the cheese, it's the crackers. Not only is the typical cracker (apart from Wasa) loaded with a lot

more calories than you would expect, but those "made with whole grain" crackers (except for Wasa) are usually a joke. The large majority of their grain content is in the form of refined flour, with a much smaller proportion coming from added whole grains. Avoid!

2. Watch out for the bread. Even whole grain bread varies from 90 calories per slice to 150 calories.

3. Fish and salads are a dieter's best friend. Look in Appendix B for more specifics.

4. Air-popped popcorn, without butter or salt, is some of the blandest solid food ever invented, but it will fill you up. The calorie contribution rounds down to zero.

5. Plan for binges! Look in the mirror, fella, and you will see a human being and not a machine. You are going to fall off the wagon. Count on it, plan for it! Binge on Wasa crackers, grapefruit, and popcorn, and laugh at your obsession. Then get right back on track.

6. Again, with apologies for the repetition: ***No alcohol, sweets, or refined flour.*** Whole grains only, and prepare to go on the wagon as it concerns alcohol. Your author grew up in Wisconsin, one of the drinkingest states in America. He is no Puritan, but he is a Midwesterner by birth and culture. "What works" is highly prized in those parts – and for this program, "what works" is ditching the beer and wine, and locking the liquor cabinet. To be honest, it was the hardest part. You have my sympathy, but make no mistake: ***You must do this. If you don't, you'll reduce your fat loss by 75%.*** This program is no day at the beach, so why not do it as quickly as you can?

7. All that label reading and calorie counting will be rewarded not just with weight loss but with a much

better diet. You will find that prepared and highly processed foods tend strongly to be more caloric, and as a result you will almost immediately switch to what you should have been eating all along.

**A Note about Women – And To Men**

This is an "Honest Diet Guide," and sometimes the truth hurts. Sorry to say, the news is not good for women. Females definitely can do this program, but in the interest of honesty, it will be more difficult than it is for men, and progress will be slower. But is that not true of every diet? Fellas, just ask her. Then listen to her about how difficult it is, because she is right as the rain. It is true for the reasons briefly given below. Spoiler: It is all about the biology.

For starters, the female body is built to store fat to a greater degree than the male body. Thus, while a good target body fat percentage is about 15% for most middle-aged men, it is in the low 20% range for most middle-aged women. This makes the "lean" idea very different for women, who face serious, demoralizing, and often conflicting social, personal, and biological pressures in this realm. For God's sake, just who in hell decided that a woman with Marilyn Monroe's body is fat? How sick is that, anyway?

More bad news on the biology front: ***Women don't need as much food as men do.*** Example: 5'8" tall, 45 years old, 160 pounds, ambulatory. That man's daily baseline calorie budget is 2,033. That woman's calorie budget is 1,825, or 10% less. Think that's rough? It gets worse when you consider that men are usually taller and heavier than women. In the United States, the average man is 5'9" tall and his average weight is 201 lbs. The average woman is 5'4" tall, and her average weight is 176 lbs. That translates to a daily calorie requirement of 2,369 for the average 45-year-old man vs. 1,888 for the average 45-year old woman, a 20% difference.

Men, if you want to know why so many women struggle so hard on the weight front, I have just told you. Now is the time to look inward and dredge up at least a tad bit of sympathy. Maybe even apologize for past cruelty? Develop some empathy, or whatever they call common decency these days.

Women, it's not all bad news. Men need to eat 8.4 fewer calories a day each year after the age of 25 because of the natural decline of metabolism with age. For women, that number is 5.8 calories. So if a man eats and exercises the same at the age of 35 as he did at the age of 25, he'll add fat at a rate of about 8-3/4 pounds per decade; if a woman does that, she'll gain at a rate of about 6 pounds per decade. (Note: It's a sliding scale, with weight gain accelerating with age on account of the ongoing natural metabolic decline. Thus, if you eat as much at age 45 as you ate at 25, with no change in exercise habits, a man will gain fat at a rate of 17 to 18 pounds per decade, and a woman at a rate of 12 pounds per decade.)

But when it comes time to lose the extra weight, she is going to have a rougher time of it for the reason I gave just above: She needs less food to begin with, so any diet will be harder for her. Again, men, would you try to remember that. And you too, women. He's probably carrying more fat, and that's no day at the beach either.

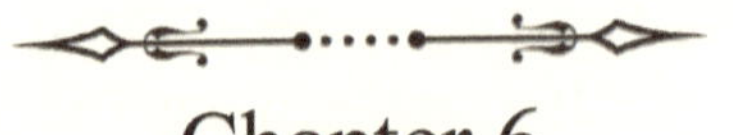

# Chapter 6
## *How This Really Works*

*Male, 52 years old, 5'11', 204 pounds, healthy. That was me.*

*Baseline calorie budget: 2,364/day*
*Cardio routine, 3x/week divided by 7: 200/day*
*Horizon: 2,564/day*
*Subtract 750/day to lose weight: 1,814/day*

Why subtract 750 calories a day? Why not 1,000 or 500? There are two answers.

First, if you lose more than 1-1/2 pounds a week, chances are that you will lose muscle along with fat. The same is true of all starvation (or "intermittent fasting") diets, and it's not a good thing.

(Exception: If you're morbidly obese and under a doctor's supervision, you will do it differently and probably put up with the muscle loss because the other problems associated with carrying WAY too much weight are critical and even life-threatening. Exercise is probably impossible, and gradualism might not be advisable. That's one reason why I'm not aiming this book at people who need to lose 100, 150, 200 or more pounds. Those situations and diets are very different, and even though the treatments bear some similarity to the material here, they are still custom-made. It would be irresponsible and dishonest to imply that this approach is the one to take.)

Back to the story. It is *hard* to deduct 750 calories a day. Because metabolism declines with age, this is especially true as you get older; it is even truer if you are female and starting from a significantly lower baseline. Frankly, I would not blame any woman (or male over about 55 years old) who deducts "only" 500 calories a day because of the difficulty of cutting more.

The flip side, of course, is that a 500-calorie reduction will work out to a pound a week and not a pound and a half. Given how restrictive – and, frankly, obsessive and generally no fun – all of this is, my attitude was to get through it as fast as possible. But I am a man, and I could eat more. In short: It is a matter of how much deprivation someone can tolerate within the maximum 750 calorie reduction limit.

**What about Other Diets?**

I have a high regard for the Atkins Diet, whose warnings about carbohydrates were prescient, and so did my long-time Harvard Medical School-educated primary care doctor. I view it as a good way to jump start the first 15 or so pounds of weight loss, but I do not see it as anything but a short-term tool. Which, by the way, is exactly why Atkins designed his "keto" diet. He wanted to prepare fat people for surgery with a quick weight loss, because fat gets in the knife's way. And yes, it works in the short term.

Something about starvation. There is a tendency of people who deploy "intermittent fasting" to simply eat more on another day – and then lie to themselves about it, typically by omission. I am skeptical of most other diets, but will note that this country's original fad diet – the "Grapefruit Diet," also called the "Hollywood Diet," popularized in the 1930s – had some merit because of the fat-burning nature of acidic foods. How much merit is anyone's guess.

The studies are not especially kind to the Grapefruit Diet. I happen to be a believer in grapefruit as a weight-loss tool, but even in the best case it is no more than an adjunct. The same goes for other diets that depict one particular food item as your savior. Forget those! Remember: No gimmicks, no miracles.

**How to measure fat? How fat to be? What's a normal weight?**

When it comes to measuring body fat, my research and practice showed that the "hydrostatic" method is by far the most accurate and consistent available to ordinary people at a reasonable price. It is done in a "dunk tank" that measures body fat by the displacement of water. In some cities, there are mobile services for this.

Second best is calipers, which measure the thickness of a pinch of skin from the midsection. Consistency is a significant issue. There are also scales that purport to measure body fat, but I found them almost laughably inconsistent. *Consumer Reports* agrees, having found that the most accurate scales are off by about 25% in either direction when purporting to measure body fat. Forget that!

The "right" body fat percentage is tricky, because the recommendations vary by sex and age. Based on research and experience, I think 15% for middle-aged men and the low 20% range for middle-aged women is a good goal. If you are too enthusiastic and go below those numbers, you might begin to look a little gaunt. The mirror is your friend, and so is the fit of your clothes. Pay attention to the numbers, but watch the mirror and feel your clothes.

For normal weights, find the Metropolitan Life Height-Weight Tables. The link is in Appendix B.

## Two Important Quirks

As you lose weight, you need fewer calories to maintain it. Thus, if you lose 20 or 40 or 60 pounds, you will be punished with a lower baseline calorie budget and the need to further reduce eating as your weight declines. It stinks, but it is not my fault! And remember: The straight-line decline in metabolism with age found by Harris and Benedict means that the older someone gets, the less they need to eat. Keep that in mind after you have lost a bunch of weight and want to keep it off.

## Will This Always Work?

Oh please! If I didn't think it would work, and if it hadn't worked for me, I wouldn't have written this book. Still: Nothing *always* works for everyone. There are some gotchas here, one being that caloric requirements are different for maintaining muscle than they are for maintaining fat. This affects a baseline calorie budget for people who are exceptionally fat or exceptionally muscular. It helps explain why I have aimed this book at the mythical "average" overweight person without any attempt to accommodate the statistical outliers. If you are in the tail of the statistical distribution, this book is probably not for you – and I suspect that you already know it.

Another possible gotcha is your level of activity. Again, I have aimed this book at the mythical average, not at people who are sick, sedentary, or bedridden, or at those in physically demanding occupations. Their calorie budgets will be lower or higher, but for most people the basic equation will work. Metabolism does vary by individual, but not by very much. If this program doesn't work, the chance that its failure is caused by your slow metabolism is extremely low. Give it two or three months, **exactly as written**. If it does not work, see Chapter 9. If it still doesn't work, then you might want to move on.

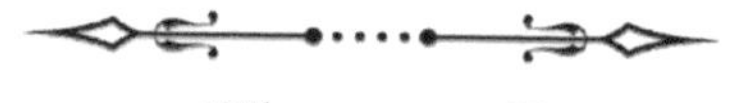

# Chapter 7
### *Tips, Tricks, Ideas, Reminders*

1. . Think you'll do it with a pill or a shot? Think again, please! One of the most popular drugs at the moment (I won't name it because I cannot afford the lawsuit) promotes a feeling of fullness, at the cost of a very long list of icky side effects.

2. If you need to feel fuller so you won't binge, I say gorge on extremely low-calorie foods instead. If anyone ever had "nausea, vomiting, diarrhea, stomach pain and constipation" from eating too many monster salads, air-popped popcorn, or Wasa crackers, I have yet to hear about it. But that's just me.

3. The drugs are the latest in a long list of illusions. In the not too distant past, some people would have doctors remove belly fat, only to find that the fat in other parts of their body – face, upper torso, back, legs, you name it – wound up taking the slack, with truly unfortunate cosmetic results. As I wrote at the outset: "no gimmicks, no magic, no shortcuts, no evasions, no secrets."

4. Start slow with the exercise. Jump into exercise too fast, and there is a high chance of quitting. If you are new to the gym or have been away for a long time, start by going once a week and working out for a half hour. Take a month to turn that into three times a week and 45 minutes per session.

5. Start fast on the new diet. Muscle fatigue is not an

issue, so there is no reason to go slow. Just do it! And remember: You are a human being not a machine. You *will* fall off the wagon. The key is what happens next: Will you give up, or will you pick yourself up, dust yourself off, and get back in the game? It really is that simple – honest.

6. ***Exercise helps, but your diet is the boss***. Take the example in Chapter 6, the 52-year-old male (the author, before implementing this program.) He cut 750 calories from his diet and burned another 200 calories a day through exercise, to lose a pound and a half a week. Only 21% of his weight loss came from exercise, while 79% came from lightening his fork and changing what was on it. If we equate this program to a dog, nutrition is the body and exercise is the tail. And we all know the old warning about not letting the tail wag the dog. The gym helps, but the cure is in the kitchen.

7. Treadmills at the gym let you dial in a desired heart rate, and walking pace. They'll adjust the angle automatically, and often have you going "uphill" to maintain your target heartbeat. The tradeoff can be that you lean forward as you walk, and strain your back doing it. You'll wind up playing with walking speed to keep the angle lower, or at least I did.

8. Keep records! Indeed, two sets of them: One to plan your diet, and the other a "before, during, after" progress report. I favor computer spreadsheets for these purposes, but there are plenty of other ways to keep track. Do not ignore this. Your progress report will become a powerful motivational tool when you are hungry and thinking about running out for a pizza.

9. Weigh yourself at the same time of day to ensure

comparability. And do not forget to measure your body fat percentage. As previously mentioned, a dunk tank is best; secondarily, calipers. No need for daily body fat measurements. Once a month will do it. As for weight, there is no need to measure daily, but the reality is that you probably will. So I will not try to convince you otherwise.

10. Your scale is only a tool, and the same goes for the numbers I've been throwing at you. Of course you should pay close attention to all of that, but in the end you will find that the mirror and the fit of your clothing will matter more than the numbers.

11. Be good to yourself. Remember, *this is an engineering problem, not a morality play*. It took a long time to get to this point, and it will take time and effort to reverse it. Do not let your progress go unnoticed by yourself, and do not forget to take satisfaction from your progress – which *will* happen if you implement this program.

12. Beware of false precision. This writer loves numbers, but that focus can go too far. For instance, should a man aim for 15% body fat, or some other percentage? Does a cardio workout have to be 45 minutes, or can it be shorter or longer? Should you exercise at 80% of maximum or something else? The answer: Just do the program as written. You will not be sorry!

13. Embrace a very big side benefit. *Because its exercise component emphasizes cardiovascular workouts, this program will significantly improve your health*. You can document this by measuring and recording your resting heart rate and blood pressure along with your body fat percentage. If you follow this

program, all three of those numbers will decline, and that will be outstanding news. Not only are you going to look better, but you are going to feel better, both physically and mentally.

28

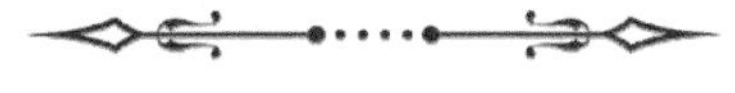

# Chapter 8
## *Puritanism, Exercise, and Diet*

Many people think that exercise is more important than it actually is in a weight-loss regime. It plays directly into the Puritan ethic that the early nutcases brought to Plymouth, Massachusetts 400 years ago. Along the way, we have translated their view of the world into all kinds of stock phrases, among them being "No pain, no gain" and "Work hard and you will succeed."

This book does something similar. Did you notice my declarations that this program is not easy? Those words were honest and true, but there is a flip side. In fact, a lot of people succeed in many ways without enduring much pain, "working hard" being a necessary but not sufficient condition for success. This country has always handed out its greatest rewards not simply for hard work but for smart work. We pay for ideas not strength, even if the two are so often seen in tandem.
A whole lot of our achievements as a society are rooted in the desire to **reduce** effort, and intelligently focus what essential efforts remain. Bottom line: Sweat to your heart's content, but do not imagine that it will get you anywhere on its own lonesome.

I remember this when I am driving out in the yonder in the summertime. I sit in my big-ass, air-conditioned, one-ton heavy-duty diesel pickup truck, the dog snoozing in the back seat. It is 102 degrees on the thermometer, and I don't care. I see the intrepid urban bicyclist vacationers in their spandex, riding uphill and imagining that there is any point to what they are doing. Have at it, I think, as I open a diet soda, crack the power windows open a tad, turn up the A/C, light a cigar, and laugh.

**My Difference: It is not your fault!**

If Puritanism was no more than exhortations to do better, it would be easier to take. But there is a flip side. It is shame, and when it comes to being overweight it goes like this: "You are fat because you are a pig." This translates into, "You are fat because you are morally defective," gluttony being one of the Seven Deadly Sins. Remember: That's not how it happened.

I offer no lectures here, other than to exhort you to keep at it. Again: ***This is an engineering problem, not a morality play.*** So quit it with the guilt and insults, and get to work. You will be glad you did, because this will work. Implement this as written and stick to it, and you will weigh less, look better, and feel better. It will take a while, because this program cuts a pound to a pound and a half a week. Trust me: It adds up. Do this exactly as written, and there is a high chance that you ***will*** succeed. You ***will*** notice, and so ***will*** others.

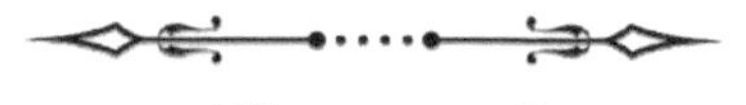

# Chapter 9
## *It's Not Working? Troubleshooting*

1. Have you given it enough time? Try it for two or three months before writing it off.

2. Did you follow it as written? As I pointed out above, guy, you are a human being, not a machine. This isn't an easy program, and you *will* fall off the wagon. When it happens, pick yourself up, dust yourself off, and get back into it. This is an "Honest Diet Guide." **You must be honest with yourself.**

3. Cornell University's calculator gives a "BMR," a basal metabolic rate. That's multiplied by 1.25 to reach a calorie budget. Maybe you need to adjust that downward and further reduce your intake.

4. Are you exercising as directed, i.e. for 45 minutes per session at a target heart rate of 220 minus your age? If not, you won't get the calorie burn that allows you to raise your calorie budget.

5. If you've **honestly** done all of the above, then move on. As I wrote earlier, nothing always works for everyone.

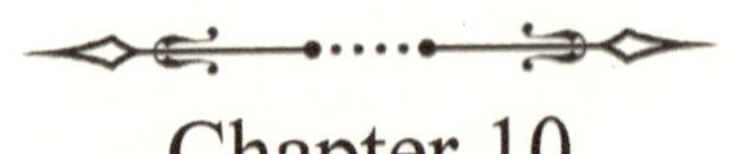

# Chapter 10
## *Composition of the American Diet,*
## *A Sad Story*

This subject would be worth another book, but I will be briefer here: Beware of modern nutritional dogma. It's a bit ironic for me to say so, given that this book rests on nutrition research. Still, the nutrition establishment made a critical, even criminal, error when so many authorities launched a war on dietary fat in the 1960s and 1970s. It continues today in the form of "low fat" foods and the carbohydrate-heavy federal food pyramid.

Food is composed of protein, carbohydrates, and fat. We need all three of them, but we've been told to reduce fat in our diet. The processed food industry has complied, and in doing so has replaced fat mostly with carbohydrates. Which, as I noted in Chapter 5, metabolizes into sugar, blocking the body's ability to consume stored fat. It also is a major contributor to diabetes, the prevalence of which increased from 0.93% of the U.S. population in 1958 to 7.4% in 2015, according to the Centers for Disease Control.

Oh, and don't confuse dietary fat with body fat, i.e. that belly roll or those thunder thighs. They are *not* the same. Eat too many calories, regardless of their composition, and you will gain body fat. Dietary fat is no more or less of a culprit on that front than carbs or protein.

**Bottom line: Don't fall for the "low fat" food illusion. Instead, focus on calories, subject to the advice in Chapter 5.**

A word or three about those new weight loss drugs. As of this writing, they are designed to fight Type 2 diabetes, and part of their mechanism is that they suppress appetite by generating a feeling of fullness. Which is what dietary fat does, only without the side effects.

You really have to hand it to Big Medical: First they pressured the government about dietary fat, so the government leaned on the food companies to reformulate their products. Then rates of diabetes and obesity went through the roof. And now Big Medical promotes the cure in the form of expensive, dangerous drugs. Guy who's reading this book, your author is grabbing your shirt, shaking you, and shouting: **Whatever else you do, get off that train, now!**

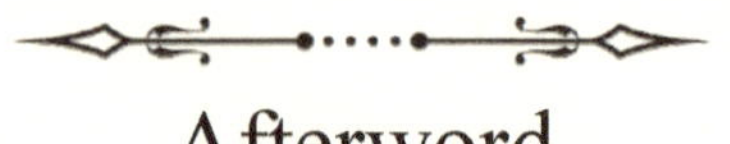

# Afterword

I have low expectations for this book's commercial success. I have only research, ethics, and personal experience to offer. I lack specific credentials in an increasingly credential-driven society. This is to be lamented, given how much of the American experience, including so many of the products and services all of us rely on, was created by the "unqualified," which is to say those without formal credentials or certifications.

To rail against mindless credentialism is to argue against a tornado, so I note it only in passing. This book is short, relatively unpadded, and isn't published by the big players. Strike one, strike two, strike three?

That much said, I based my successful weight loss effort, and later this book, on *highly credentialed* sources. I listed them in Appendix A, and invite close scrutiny. This book makes me the cook, not the farmer, the processor, the food regulator, or the grocery store. Yet, remember this: without the cook, there's no meal. My role here has been to combine ingredients into an appealing, digestible whole. *Bon appétit!*

If the gods of life's roulette wheel are smiling and this book gets the attention it deserves, not only will I be pleasantly shocked but there will be much nitpicking. Most of it will be driven by jealousy and will amount to nothing. If that turns out to be wrong and there are errors, I will change the next version to incorporate any valid, material objections.

Again, though, as I write I expect this little tome to vanish into obscurity, even though it should not. To the contrary, if "the masses" were to become familiar with what I have written, we would have a far less obese and unhealthy population. Oh well. That's the way the fattening cookie crumbles.

I want to give credit not only to Harris and Benedict, whose research formed the foundation of this book, but to a most unlikely source: The L.A. Fitness chain of gyms, where I learned of their research to begin with.

When I joined L.A. Fitness in Seattle in the early years of the 21st century, my membership included a workbook. In the back of that book, there was the Harris-Benedict formula. I was intrigued, so I gave it a try. But it did not work as well I expected, and that puzzled me. I looked harder and discovered that the formula was mis-transcribed. Someone had switched a mathematical sign, and the error was worth a half a pound a week's worth of overeating. I called their corporate headquarters and left a brief voicemail message that I'd found a significant error, and that if anyone cared they could call me.

I didn't expect a return call, but three weeks later it came. I asked the caller to grab the workbook, sit at a computer, and call up Cornell University's website. I patiently took them through the correct formula vs. the one they had published. If L.A. Fitness had thought highly enough of the Harris-Benedict equation to include it in its workbook, I said, why not get it right? The caller agreed, and about a month later I saw a pallet of new workbooks at my location. Someone cared enough to correct the mistake, surely at material expense. Kudos to L.A. Fitness for introducing me to Harris and Benedict, and kudos to them for not ignoring my call but instead for correcting their error. Integrity, it's what's for breakfast.

36

# Appendix A
## Data & Sources

**The Harris-Benedict Equation, raw formula**

Men: 66.5 + (13.75 x kg weight) + (5.003 x cm height) - (6.775 x age)

Women: 655.1 + (9.563 x kg weight) + (1.850 x cm height) - (4.676 x age)

Multiply the results by 1.25 for the daily caloric requirement.

**The Harris-Benedict Equation, online**

https://www.ncbi.nlm.nih.gov/pmc/articles/PMC1091498/

https://bmicalc.org/resources/harris-benedict-equation

bit.ly/hbiomet

*A Biometric Study of Basal Metabolism in Man*, 1919
By J. Arthur Harris and Francis G. Benedict
Carnegie Institution of Washington, 1919
re-published by Google Books

## Calories and Exercise

These are per-hour numbers. Note that the machines in gyms will calculate the calorie expenditures for you.

296 – Aerobics, high impact
354 – Bicycling, 10-12 mph (light)
473 – Bicycling, 12-4 mph (moderate)
591 – Bicycling, 14-16 mph (vigorous)
324 – Bicycling, stationary, 100 watts (light)
413 – Bicycling, stationary, 150 watts (moderate)
619 – Bicycling, stationary, 200 watts (vigorous)
473 – Rope jumping (slow)
591 – Rope jumping (moderate)
708 – Rope jumping (fast)
473 – Running, 5 mph (12 min./mile)
738 – Running, 7.5 mph (8 min./mile)
945 – Running, 10 mph (6 min/mile)
354 – Swimming (leisurely, not lap swimming, general)
473 – Swimming (laps, freestyle, moderate)
591 – Swimming (laps, freestyle, fast, vigorous)
206 – Walking, 3.0 mph (level, moderate)
236 – Walking, 3.5 mph (level, brisk)
266 – Walking, 4.0 mph (level, very brisk)
236 – Water aerobics/calisthenics
473 – Circuit training, elevated pulse rate, vigorous
354 – Stair treadmill/elliptical trainer, general
561 – Ski machine, general
206 – Rowing, stationary, 50 watts (light)
413 – Rowing, stationary, 100 watts (moderate)
501 – Rowing, stationary, 150 watts (vigorous)
177 – Weightlifting, free weights or machine (light to moderate)
354 – Weightlifting, free weights or machine (vigorous)

**Workout methodology: Maximum heart rate, duration**

https://www.cdc.gov/physicalactivity/basics/measuring/heartrate.htm

https://www.bodybuilding.com/fun/calhr.htm

https://www.bodybuilding.com/fun/betteru16.htm

**Correct body fat percentage goal**

https://www.dexafit.com/blog2/what-is-the-ideal-body-fat-percentage

https://www.newhealthadvisor.org/Body-Fat-Percentage-Chart.html

**How to measure body fat**

https://www.healthline.com/nutrition/ways-to-measure-body-fat

https://www.bodybuilding.com/content/how-to-measure-your-body-fat.html

https://www.medicalnewstoday.com/articles/body-fat-scale-accuracy

**Evaluation of the "grapefruit diet"**

https://www.everydayhealth.com/diet-nutrition/grapefruit-diet.aspx

**Muscle loss from starvation diets**

https://www.gq.com/story/calorie-weight-loss

https://inbodyusa.com/blogs/inbodyblog/what-happens-to-your-body-composition-when-you-starve-to-lose-weight/

https://www.nia.nih.gov/health/calorie-restriction-and-fasting-diets-what-do-we-know

**Calories in a pound of fat**

https://www.caloriesecrets.net/how-many-calories-are-in-a-pound-of-body-fat/

**Metabolism of alcohol**

https://pubmed.ncbi.nlm.nih.gov/16047538/

https://www.ncbi.nlm.nih.gov/books/NBK22524/

https://www.ncbi.nlm.nih.gov/pmc/articles/PMC3484320/

https://www.ncbi.nlm.nih.gov/pmc/articles/PMC2493591/

**Metabolism of carbohydrates and diabetes link**

https://healthyeating.sfgate.com/steps-digestion-carbohydrates-4053.html

https://healthyeating.sfgate.com/whole-grains-difficult-digest-10781.html

https://steptohealth.com/7-negative-effects-refined-flour/

https://academic.oup.com/jn/article/137/4/923/4664712

## Height & Weight Information

https://www.cdc.gov/nchs/data/nhsr/nhsr122-508.pdf

http://www.assessmentpsychology.com/metlife.htm

## Obesity and Diabetes: Historical Prevalence

https://usafacts.org/articles/obesity-rate-nearly-triples-united-states-over-last-50-years/

https://www.cdc.gov/diabetes/statistics/slides/long_term_trends.pdf

## The war on dietary fat

https://pubmed.ncbi.nlm.nih.gov/24911982/

https://blog.perfectsnacks.com/the-war-on-fat/

https://openheart.bmj.com/content/2/1/e000196?ijkey=fc62393f54b48911eb6c4bcf3fb5a5355ecf196e&keytype2=tf_ipsecsha

# Appendix B
*Calories in common foods*

Many readings depend on the size of the item, so consider these approximations for many items, rounded to the nearest 5 calories.

https://www.calories.info + miscellaneous credible sources.

**Meat & Fish**

Fish, broiled Halibut: 35/oz

Chicken breast: 50/oz, with skin, 40/oz without

Beef steak: 70/oz

Pork roast: 80/oz

Cold Cuts/Lunch Meat: 30-100/slice, typically 50.

Turkey, roast: 60/oz.

Smoked salmon: 35/oz

Tuna canned in water: 75/oz

Ground beef, 90% lean: 50/oz

**Starches**

Spaghetti, cooked: 220/cup

Bread: 90-150/slice, typically 110.

English Muffin: 130

Other Muffins: 160-210

Hot Dog Bun: 120

Hamburger Bun: 140 calories

Crackers: Club brand, 140/oz. Wheat Thins, 135/oz. Wasa, 70/oz

Potatoes: 30/oz

Potato chips: Kettle brand, 140/oz

**Fast Food, Snacks & Sweets**

Pizza: 80-100/slice
Big Mac: 560/sandwich

McDonald's cheeseburger: 300/sandwich

McRib: 450/sandwich

Burger King Whopper: 670/sandwich

Mac & Cheese: 350/cup

Oreos: 55/cookie

Nestle Toll House chocolate chip: 105/cookie

Pretzels: 110/oz

**Breakfast**

Cereal: 140/1.5 cup serving of Cheerios, not incl. milk.

Bacon: 45/slice

Eggs: 80

Pancakes: 95 for a medium size.

Syrup: 215/quarter-cup, maple.

Sausage link: 90 per link, pork.

Author's "Power Breakfast": 2 slices whole-wheat toast, 2 oz smoked salmon, 1 oz cream cheese, 4 medium-sized carrots (peeled and juiced), 1 apple or orange (juiced), ginger, 600

**Condiments**

Peanut Butter: 170/oz

Cream Cheese (full fat): 110/oz

Butter: 100/ tblsp

Mayonnaise: 90/tblsp, full fat

Salad dressing: 85/tblsp, full fat

Cheese, cheddar: 115/oz

Cheese, American: 40/slice

**Fruits & Veggies**

Apples, oranges, pears, bananas: 90.

Lettuce: 5/cup

**Drinks**

Wine: 125/5-1/2 oz glass

Beer: 155/12 oz

Liquor: 100/1.5 oz shot

Milk (whole, 3.25% fat): 160/cup

Soda w/Sugar: 170/12 oz

Juices, store-bought: 15-20/oz

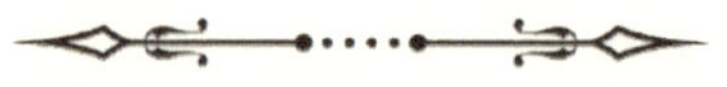

# About the Author
*Who is this guy, anyway?*

Charles Pluckhahn is retired from two careers, one as a newspaper journalist when that business still had high standards pertaining to facts, balance, ethics, and the pursuit of objectivity, and the second in finance, where he occasionally claimed to be "the only honest securities analyst you will ever meet."

In the first career, he was a general assignment and business reporter for the Dubuque, Iowa *Telegraph Herald*; a labor reporter for the *Kansas City Star*; and opened the Washington, D.C. bureau of *Investor's Daily* (later *Investor's Business Daily*), where he spent five years covering various political and financial issues, including Federal Reserve policy.

In the second career, he was a securities analyst and portfolio manager for State Street Research and Management Co., one of Boston's first mutual and pension fund managers. Later, he was a telecommunications analyst, covering broadband equipment and services companies for two regional investment banks, Dain Rauscher Wessels and Stephens Inc., and served on the board of directors for a telecommunications equipment startup.

He earned a B.A. degree from the University of Wisconsin-Madison in 1979, and an MBA from the University of Pennsylvania's Wharton School of

Business in 1990.

After getting fat from the combination of investment luches and dinners, and declining metabolism, he struggled to button his pants and realized that he'd reached a decision point. Would he become obese, or not? He chose to face facts did a lot of research, and faced the facts. He wrote this book to show readers how they can do the same thing and win the battle.